Knockdown That Breast Cancer:

A Complete Guide to Preventing, Treating, and Conquering Breast Cancer

By

Rosie J. Mullen

TABLE OF CONTENT

Introduction

Knockdown That Breast Cancer is a comprehensive guide to the prevention, diagnosis, and treatment of breast cancer. Written for those who have been diagnosed with the disease, those at risk of developing it, and those who want to learn more about it, the book provides up-to-date information about the latest medical advances, treatments, and lifestyle choices.

The book begins with an overview of the disease, including its causes and risk factors. It then explores the various types of breast cancer, the diagnostic tests and treatments available, and the available treatments for each type. It also covers the emotional and psychological aspects of living with the disease, as well as the importance of support and lifestyle changes.

Knock Down That Breast Cancer is written in a straightforward, easy-to-understand style that makes it accessible to readers of all levels of understanding. The book is filled with helpful tips, resources, and advice to help readers make informed decisions about their health and well-being. It also includes a cookbook for the treatment of breast cancer, With this book as a companion, readers can take charge of their treatment and find the strength to face their breast cancer with confidence.

CHAPTER 1

Overview of breast cancer

Breast Cancer

Breast Cancer is usually a malignant tumor that develops from the lining of the milk ducts or the lobules that supply the ducts with milk. Breast cancer can spread to other parts of the body and is the most common cancer among women in the United States.

The most common type of breast cancer is ductal carcinoma, which originates in the cells of the milk ducts. Other types include lobular carcinoma, which starts in the lobules, and inflammatory breast cancer, which is an aggressive form of breast cancer that causes the breast to become red and swollen.

In its early stages, breast cancer may not cause any symptoms, but as it progresses, a lump or thickening in the breast may be felt. Other symptoms include changes in the skin of the breast, such as dimpling or puckering, nipple discharge or retraction, and pain in the breast or armpit.

Testing for breast cancer may include a physical exam of the breast, a mammogram, an ultrasound, an MRI, and a biopsy. Treatment for breast cancer may include surgery, radiation therapy, chemotherapy, hormone therapy, and targeted therapy.

Stages and Grades of Breast Cancer

Stages of Breast Cancer

Breast cancer is typically diagnosed in stages, ranging from stage 0 (also known as carcinoma in situ) to stage IV (also known as advanced or metastatic cancer).

Stage 0: In stage 0, the cancer cells are limited to the inner lining of the breast ducts and have not spread outside the ducts.

Stage I: In stage I, the cancer cells are still contained within the breast and may or may not have spread to the lymph nodes in the armpit.

Stage II: In stage II, the cancer cells have spread to the lymph nodes in the armpit or to nearby tissues in the breast.

Stage III: In stage III, the cancer cells have spread to the chest wall, skin of the breast, or other organs in the chest.

Stage IV: In stage IV, the cancer cells have spread to other parts of the body such as the lungs, liver, brain, or bones

Grades of Breast Cancer

Breast cancer is typically classified into four grades, based on the appearance of the cancer cells under a microscope.

Grade 1 (low-grade): This type of breast cancer is often referred to as "well-differentiated," meaning that the cancer cells look very much like normal cells, and tend to grow and spread more slowly.

Grade 2 (intermediate-grade): This type of breast cancer is referred to as "moderately-differentiated," meaning that the cancer cells look less like normal cells than Grade 1, but more like normal cells than Grade 3.

This type of breast cancer tends to grow and spread more quickly than in Grade 1.

Grade 3 (high-grade): This type of breast cancer is referred to as "poorly-differentiated," meaning that the cancer cells look very different from normal cells and tend to grow and spread more quickly.

Grade 4 (undifferentiated): This type of breast cancer is referred to as "undifferentiated," meaning that the cancer cells look very different from normal cells and tend to grow and spread very quickly.

The grade of breast cancer helps to determine the treatment plan, as well as the prognosis. Low-grade cancers tend to have a better prognosis than high-grade cancers, and the treatments may vary depending on the grade of cancer.

Types and Subtypes of Breast Cancer

Types of Breast Cancer

It is the most common cancer among women in the United States and the second most common cancer overall.

There are several types of breast cancer, depending on the type of cells affected.

• Ductal Carcinoma: This is the most common type of breast cancer, accounting for 80% of all breast cancers. It starts in the cells of the ducts, which are the passages that carry milk from the lobules to the nipple.

• Lobular Carcinoma: This is the second most common type of breast cancer, accounting for 10-15% of all breast cancers. It starts in the cells of the lobules, which are the glands that make milk.

• Inflammatory Breast Cancer: This is a rare but aggressive type of breast cancer that accounts for 1-5% of all breast cancers. It is characterized by redness, swelling, and warmth in the breast, as well as a dimpled or pitted appearance of the skin.

• Paget's Disease: This is a rare type of breast cancer that affects the nipple and areola, accounting for 1-4% of all breast cancers. It is characterized by a scaly, red rash around the nipple and areola that can be itchy and tender.

• Phyllodes Tumors: This is a rare type of breast cancer that accounts for less than 1% of all breast cancers. It is characterized by a rapidly growing, benign tumor that forms in the connective tissue of the breast.

No matter what type of breast cancer you have, it is important to get prompt treatment to have the best chance of recovery.

Subtypes of Breast Cancer

There are several subtypes of breast cancer, each with different characteristics and treatments. The most common subtypes are:

1. Invasive Ductal Carcinoma (IDC): This is the most common type of breast cancer, accounting for about 80% of all breast cancer cases.

 It begins in the cells of the milk ducts, then spreads through the breast tissue to other parts of the body. Treatment typically includes surgery, radiation, and/or chemotherapy.

2. Invasive Lobular Carcinoma (ILC): This type of breast cancer begins in the milk-producing glands (lobules) and can spread outside the breast. Treatment typically includes surgery, radiation, and/or chemotherapy.

3. Triple-Negative Breast Cancer: This type of breast cancer is characterized by the absence of three proteins (estrogen, progesterone, and HER2/neu) that are typically found in other types of breast cancer. Treatment typically includes surgery, radiation, and/or chemotherapy.

4. Inflammatory Breast Cancer: This is a rare and aggressive type of breast cancer. The breast appears red, swollen, and warm to the touch. Treatment typically includes surgery, radiation, and/or chemotherapy.

5. Metastatic Breast Cancer: This type of breast cancer has spread from the original tumor site to other parts of the body, such as the bones, liver, brain, or lungs.

Treatment typically includes chemotherapy and/or targeted therapies.

CHAPTER 2

Causes of Breast Cancer

The Genetics of Breast Cancer

Breast cancer is the most common type of cancer in women and can be caused by a variety of factors, including genetic factors.

Genetic mutations in certain genes can increase the risk of developing breast cancer. Mutations in either of these genes increase the risk of breast cancer in women by about five times compared to women in the general population. In addition, mutations in these genes can also increase the risk of developing other types of cancers, such as ovarian and prostate cancer.

Other genes, such as TP53 and PTEN, can also increase the risk of breast cancer. Mutations in these genes can increase the risk of developing breast cancer by up to five times compared to those without mutations.

In addition to mutations in these genes, certain environmental factors can also increase the risk of breast cancer. These include exposure to certain hormones, such as those found in hormone replacement therapy, and radiation exposure.

Overall, genetic mutations in certain genes can increase the risk of developing breast cancer significantly. It is important to know your family history and to talk to your doctor about genetic testing if you are at an increased risk of developing breast cancer.

The Environmental Causes of Breast Cancer.

The environmental causes of breast cancer are numerous and complex. Exposure to environmental pollutants such as chemicals, radiation, and lifestyle factors can all increase the risk of breast cancer.

Chemical pollutants, such as pesticides, industrial solvents, and air pollution, release carcinogenic compounds that can enter the body and increase breast cancer risk. Radiation exposure, both through medical imaging and environmental sources, can also increase risk.

Lifestyle factors, such as dietary choices, physical activity, alcohol consumption, and smoking, also affect breast cancer risk. Diets high in processed foods and red meat, low in fruits and vegetables, and low in fiber, increase the risk of breast cancer. Physical inactivity, alcohol consumption, and smoking all increase risk as well.

Finally, certain hormone-disrupting chemicals, such as bisphenol A (BPA), phthalates, and parabens, have been linked to an increased risk of breast cancer. These chemicals, found in many everyday products, can disrupt the body's natural hormone balance and increase breast cancer risk.

Overall, the environmental causes of breast cancer are complex and interrelated. Reducing exposure to environmental pollutants and maintaining a healthy lifestyle can help reduce risk.

The Hormonal Causes of Breast Cancer

Breast cancer is a condition that can be caused by several different factors, including genetic mutations, environmental exposures, lifestyle factors, and hormonal influences. Hormonal influences are believed to be one of the main causes of breast cancer, as high levels of certain hormones in the body can increase the risk of developing the disease.

Estrogen is the primary hormone that is believed to be linked to breast cancer. When levels of estrogen are too high, it can lead to an increased risk of developing the disease. This can be due to an increase in the body's production of estrogen, or it can be due to the body being exposed to external sources of estrogen, such as hormone replacement therapy or certain forms of birth control.

Progesterone is another hormone that is believed to be involved in breast cancer. This hormone helps to regulate the menstrual cycle and is believed to be linked to the development of certain types of breast cancer.

High levels of progesterone can also increase the risk of developing breast cancer, as this hormone can stimulate the growth of breast cells that are already abnormal.

Finally, insulin is a hormone that is believed to be linked to breast cancer. Insulin is a hormone that helps regulate the body's blood sugar levels, and high levels of insulin can increase the risk of developing the disease. This can be due to an increase in the body's production of insulin, or it can be due to the body being exposed to external sources of insulin, such as certain medications or diets that are high in sugar.

CHAPTER 3

Diagnosis and Treatment

Early Detection and Diagnosis of Breast Cancer

Early detection and diagnosis of breast cancer are important for improving the chances of successful treatment. The most common diagnostic tests for breast cancer are mammograms and biopsies.

Mammograms

Mammograms are X-ray images of the breast that can detect changes in the tissue and can be used to diagnose breast cancer. Mammograms can detect tumors that may not be felt by physical examination. Regular screening mammograms are recommended for women over age 40 and may begin as early as age 35 for those at high risk for breast cancer.

Biopsies

 A biopsy is a procedure in which a sample of the suspicious tissue is removed and examined for the presence of cancer cells. A biopsy can be done on a suspicious lump or area identified on a mammogram. The type of biopsy performed depends on the location of the suspicious area and the size of the tumor.

If the biopsy results are positive for cancer, further tests may be done to determine the stage of cancer, which will help guide treatment.

Symptoms of Breast Cancer

Breast cancer is a type of cancer that begins in the cells of the breast. Symptoms of breast cancer vary from person to person and may include:

1. A lump or thickening in the breast, armpit, or around the collarbone

2. Changes in the size, shape, or feel of the breast

3. A change in the look or feel of the skin on the breast, such as puckering, dimpling, or redness

4. Nipple discharge, particularly if it is bloody

5. A retracted nipple or a change in the direction of the nipple

6. Pain in the breast or armpit

7. Swelling in the armpit or around the collarbone

These symptoms do not always mean that a person has breast cancer. It is important to speak to a doctor about any changes that are noticed. A doctor can determine if the symptoms are due to cancer or another condition.

Natural Treatment for Breast Cancer

Natural treatments for breast cancer are therapies that are non-invasive and used to support traditional medical approaches to treatment. Natural treatments include herbal remedies and supplements.

Herbal Remedies for Breast Cancer Treatment

Herbal remedies have been used in traditional medicine for centuries as a way to treat a variety of health issues, including breast cancer. Many herbs and natural remedies have been studied for their potential to help reduce the risk of developing breast cancer.

Green tea is one of the most studied herbal remedies for breast cancer. Studies have shown that compounds in green tea have powerful antioxidant and anti-inflammatory properties that may help protect against certain forms of cancer.

Astragalus, Studies have found that compounds in astragalus may help inhibit the growth of breast cancer cells and can also help reduce inflammation. Additionally, astragalus may help reduce the side effects of chemotherapy and radiation therapy.

Turmeric is another herb that has been used for centuries in traditional Indian medicine. Studies have found that compounds in turmeric called curcuminoids may help reduce inflammation and may help inhibit the growth of breast cancer cells. Additionally, turmeric may help reduce the side effects of chemotherapy and radiation therapy.

Ginger is another herb that has been studied for its potential to help in the treatment of breast cancer. Research has found that compounds in ginger may help reduce inflammation, inhibit the growth of cancer cells, and may even help reduce the side effects of chemotherapy and radiation therapy.

Herbal remedies may be beneficial in the treatment of breast cancer, but they should not be used as a substitute for conventional treatments.

It is important to talk to your doctor before using any herbal remedies to ensure that they will not interfere with any medications or treatments you are currently taking. Additionally, it is important to remember that herbal remedies have not been evaluated or approved by the FDA, so their effectiveness and safety may not be known.

Supplement for the Treatment of Breast Cancer

Breast cancer is a type of cancer that affects the breast tissue, and can be both invasive and noninvasive. Treatment options for breast cancer can vary depending on the type and stage of cancer.

Supplements are sometimes recommended as part of a breast cancer treatment plan. Some of the most common supplements include omega-3 fatty acids, vitamin D, and curcumin. They may help reduce inflammation, which is associated with cancer and may also reduce the risk of recurrence after initial treatment.

Vitamin D is an important part of the body's natural defense against cancer.

Vitamin D helps regulate the growth of cells and may reduce the risk of certain cancers, including breast cancer.

Curcumin is a compound found in turmeric, a spice commonly used in Indian cooking. Curcumin has been found to have anti-inflammatory, antioxidant, and anti-cancer properties. It may help reduce the risk of recurrence after initial treatment and slow the growth of cancer cells.

These supplements, when taken in recommended amounts, can be beneficial for breast cancer patients. However, it is important to talk to your doctor before taking any supplements, as some supplements may interact with other medications or treatments.

Modern Treatment Options

Modern treatment for breast cancer typically consists of surgery, radiation therapy, hormone therapy, and/or chemotherapy. Depending on the stage of cancer, one or more of these treatments may be recommended.

Surgery Treatment for Breast Cancer

Breast cancer surgery is a common type of treatment for many forms of breast cancer. Depending on the type and stage of breast cancer, different surgical techniques are used.

A lumpectomy or partial mastectomy is a type of minimally invasive breast surgery. This type of surgery removes the tumor and a small amount of surrounding tissue. It is usually used for smaller tumors in the early stages of breast cancer.

A mastectomy is typically recommended for larger tumors or advanced stages of breast cancer. A mastectomy may also be recommended if there is a high risk of cancer coming back after a lumpectomy.

Sentinel node biopsy is a procedure used to determine if cancer has spread to the lymph nodes. A sentinel node biopsy involves removing a few of the lymph nodes closest to the tumor to test for cancer cells.

Breast reconstruction surgery is a type of surgery rebuilds the breast using implants or tissue from another part of the body. It can help women who have had a mastectomy restore their appearance and body image.

Benefits of surgical treatment of breast cancer

1. Improved survival rates: Surgery is one of the most common treatments for breast cancer and is often the most effective option for removing cancerous tissue. In many cases, surgery can improve survival rates for people with early-stage breast cancer and can be used to prevent the spread of cancer cells to other parts of the body.

2. Improved quality of life: Surgery can help improve a person's quality of life post-treatment by providing relief from symptoms like pain and fatigue. Surgery can also help reduce the risk of recurrence and the need for additional treatments.

3. Improved cosmetic results: Depending on the type of surgery, some people may experience improved cosmetic results after treatment. For example, breast reconstruction can help restore the appearance of the breasts after a mastectomy.

4. Prevention of cancer spread: Surgery is often used to remove cancerous tissue and prevent it from spreading to other parts of the body. This can help reduce the risk of metastasis and improve the overall prognosis.

5. Improved access to other treatments: Surgery can be used to remove cancerous tissue, making it easier for people to access other treatments such as chemotherapy or radiation. This can help improve the effectiveness of other treatments and reduce the risk of recurrence.

Surgery is one of the most common treatments for breast cancer, to remove the tumor and any cancerous cells. While the procedure can be successful in treating the disease, it can also cause a range of side effects.

The most common side effects of breast cancer surgery include pain, swelling, and fatigue. Pain is often managed with medications, but it may be difficult to manage if the surgery was extensive. Swelling can occur in the operated area and may last for several weeks. Fatigue is a common side effect of any surgery, and it may take several days or weeks to recover.

Other possible side effects of surgery for breast cancer include infection and scarring. Infections can occur when bacteria enter the surgical wound, and they can be treated with antibiotics. Scarring can occur as a result of the surgery and may be permanent.

Some more serious side effects, such as lymphedema, can also occur after breast cancer surgery. Lymphedema is a condition in which fluid accumulates in the arms, chest or other parts of the body due to the disruption of the lymphatic system. Lymphedema can cause discomfort, swelling, and infection, and it can be managed with a range of treatments, including massage, compression garments, and exercise.

Finally, some people may experience emotional side effects after breast cancer surgery, such as anxiety, depression, and a loss of self-confidence. These feelings can be managed with counselling, support groups, and medications.

Overall, while there are potential side effects associated with breast cancer surgery, they can usually be managed with medications and other treatments.

It is important to talk to your doctor about any concerns you have regarding the potential side effects of surgery so that you can receive the proper treatment.

Radiation therapy for breast cancer treatment

Radiation therapy is a type of treatment that uses high-energy radiation to destroy cancer cells and shrink tumors. It is commonly used to treat breast cancer and is an important part of both curative and palliative treatments.

Radiation therapy works by damaging the DNA in cancer cells, which prevents them from growing and dividing. As the radiation passes through the body, it also damages healthy cells, but they are usually able to repair themselves. The radiation is targeted to specific areas to minimize the damage to healthy tissue.

The most common type of radiation therapy used to treat breast cancer is external beam radiation therapy. This type of radiation is delivered from a machine outside the body and is often combined with other treatments, such as surgery and chemotherapy.

Radiation therapy can be used before or after surgery or in combination with chemotherapy. It may also be used as part of an adjuvant therapy, which is used to reduce the risk of cancer recurrence.

During radiation therapy, the patient will lie on a treatment table and a radiation technician will use a device to precisely aim the radiation at the tumor. Treatment sessions typically last from 10 to 30 minutes and are usually given five days a week for five to seven weeks.

Radiation therapy is an important part of treating breast cancer and can be used to cure, shrink, or slow the growth of tumors.

Major Benefits of Radiation Therapy for the Treatment of Breast Cancer

Radiation therapy (also known as radiotherapy) is a common treatment for breast cancer. It can be used to destroy cancer cells in the breast, as well as any cancer cells that may have spread to other parts of the body.

1. Effective Treatment: Radiation therapy is an effective treatment for early-stage breast cancer, as well as a complement to other treatments like surgery or chemotherapy. Studies have found that radiation therapy can reduce the risk of cancer recurrence and improve survival rates.

2. Minimally Invasive: Radiation therapy is a relatively painless and non-invasive treatment option. Unlike surgery, radiation therapy is done externally, meaning it does not require any incisions or anesthetic. This makes

it a good choice for people who cannot tolerate surgery or prefer a less invasive treatment.

3. Targeted Treatment: Radiation therapy is a targeted treatment, meaning it can be used to accurately target and destroy cancer cells in the breast without damaging healthy tissue. This makes it a safe and effective treatment for breast cancer.

4. Improved Quality of Life: Radiation therapy can help improve the quality of life for people with breast cancer. It can reduce pain and other symptoms associated with the disease, as well as reduce the risk of cancer recurrence, allowing patients to live longer and healthier lives.

Overall, radiation therapy can be an effective and safe treatment option for breast cancer. It can help reduce the risk of cancer recurrence and improve the quality of life for patients, making it a good choice for many people.

Major side effects of radiation therapy for breast cancer treatment

Radiation therapy is an important treatment option for many people with breast cancer. It helps to destroy cancer cells in the breast and can reduce the risk of cancer returning. However, like any medical treatment, radiation therapy can cause side effects.

Common side effects of radiation therapy for breast cancer include fatigue, skin changes, breast swelling, and breast tenderness.

Fatigue: Fatigue is a common side effect of radiation therapy and can vary in severity from person to person. It may begin during the first few weeks of treatment and can last for several weeks or months after treatment is finished.

Skin changes: Radiation therapy can cause the skin in the treatment area to become dry, itchy, and red. In some cases, the skin may become darker or more sensitive to the touch.

Breast swelling: Radiation therapy can cause the breast to swell, which can cause discomfort or pain.

Breast tenderness: Radiation therapy can cause the breast to become tender and sensitive to the touch. This can last for several weeks after treatment is finished.

Other possible side effects of radiation therapy may include nausea, hair loss, and changes in the breast shape or size. It is important to speak to your doctor about any side effects you are experiencing.

Hormone Therapy for Breast Cancer Treatment

Hormone therapy, also known as endocrine therapy, is a type of breast cancer treatment that works by either blocking hormones from interacting with cancer cells or reducing the production of hormones that help cancer cells grow.

It is most often used to treat hormone receptor-positive (HR+) breast cancer, which means cancer cells that rely on hormones to grow.

Hormone therapy usually involves taking medications such as tamoxifen, anastrozole, letrozole, fulvestrant, exemestane, or other hormone therapy drugs. These medications can be taken orally or intravenously and can be used alone or in combination with other treatments, such as chemotherapy or radiation.

Hormone therapy works by blocking the hormones estrogen and progesterone from attaching to cancer cells. Without these hormones, the cancer cells can no longer grow or spread. Hormone therapy can also reduce the production of hormones, including estrogen and testosterone, which can help slow or stop the growth of cancer cells.

Hormone therapy is typically used to treat advanced stages of HR+ breast cancer. It can also be used to reduce the risk of recurrence in women who have already been treated for HR+ breast cancer. It is important to note that hormone therapy is not a cure for breast cancer, but it can help slow the growth of cancer cells and reduce the risk of recurrence.

The major benefits of hormonal therapy for breast cancer treatment

Hormonal therapy is a type of treatment for breast cancer that involves the use of medications to block the effects of hormones in the body. It is used to treat cancers that are sensitive to hormones, such as hormone receptor-positive breast cancers, and to reduce the risk of recurrence after surgery and other treatments.

The major benefits of hormonal therapy for breast cancer treatment include:

1. Improved survival rates: Hormonal therapy has been shown to improve survival rates for women with hormone-sensitive breast cancers. Studies have shown that women who received hormonal therapy after surgery for early-stage breast cancer had improved overall survival rates compared to those who did not receive the treatment.

2. Reduces risk of recurrence: Hormonal therapy can reduce the risk of recurrence after surgery and other treatments for breast cancer.

This is especially important for women who have hormone-sensitive breast cancers, as these cancers are more likely to recur.

3. Reduced side effects: Hormonal therapy is generally well tolerated and has fewer side effects than chemotherapy and other treatments. The most common side effects include hot flashes, vaginal dryness, and mood changes.

4. Better quality of life: Hormonal therapy can improve quality of life by reducing symptoms of breast cancer and its treatment. For example, it can reduce pain and discomfort associated with cancer, such as breast pain and tenderness.

 Hormonal therapy is an important treatment option for women with hormone-sensitive breast cancers. It can improve survival rates, reduce the risk of recurrence, and improve quality of life. However, it is important to discuss the potential risks and benefits with your doctor before starting hormonal therapy.

Major Side Effects of Hormone Therapy for Breast Cancer Treatment

Hormone therapy is a type of treatment for breast cancer that involves blocking the effect of hormones like estrogen and progesterone that can fuel the growth of some breast cancer cells. While hormone therapy can be a highly effective treatment for breast cancer, it is important to understand that it can cause serious side effects which includes:

• Hot flashes and night sweats: These are common side effects of hormone therapy and can occur due to changes in the levels of hormones in the body.

• Vaginal dryness and itching: Hormone therapy can cause the walls of the vagina to become thin and dry, leading to itching and burning sensations.

• Mood swings: Hormone therapy can cause hormonal fluctuations that can result in mood changes.

• Weight gain: Hormone therapy can cause an increase in appetite, leading to weight gain.

• Bone loss: Hormone therapy can cause a decrease in bone mineral density, leading to an increased risk of fractures.

• Fatigue: Hormone therapy can cause a decrease in energy levels, leading to fatigue.

• Increased risk of blood clots: Hormone therapy can increase the risk of developing blood clots.

• Increased risk of stroke: Hormone therapy can increase the risk of stroke, especially in women who already have other risk factors for stroke.

Increased risk of heart attack: Hormone therapy can increase the risk of a heart attack.

• Increased risk of cancer: Hormone therapy can increase the risk of developing certain types of cancer, such as uterine cancer.

Chemotherapy treatment for breast cancer

Chemotherapy is usually given as an intravenous (IV) infusion, which means the drugs are delivered directly into a vein. The type of chemotherapy and the combination of drugs used will depend on the type and stage of cancer.

The most common drugs used to treat breast cancer are doxorubicin (Adriamycin), cyclophosphamide (Cytoxan), paclitaxel (Taxol), and 5-fluorouracil (5-FU). These drugs are usually given in combination with other drugs.

The goal of chemotherapy is to kill cancer cells that may have spread to other parts of the body. It can also shrink tumors and reduce symptoms. However, chemotherapy can also cause side effects, such as fatigue, nausea, hair loss, and an increased risk of infection.

Patients receiving chemotherapy may also be given supportive medications to help reduce the side effects.

These medications can include anti-nausea drugs, steroids, and growth factors like filgrastim (Neupogen) to help boost the immune system.

Chemotherapy is usually given in cycles of treatment, which may last for several weeks. The number of cycles and the length of treatment will depend on the type of cancer and the patient's overall health.

Chemotherapy is an important part of cancer treatment, and it can be a very effective way to treat breast cancer.

The major benefits of chemotherapy treatments for breast cancer

Chemotherapy is a common treatment for breast cancer, and can be used alone or in combination with other treatments such as surgery and radiation therapy.

The main benefits of chemotherapy for breast cancer are that it can reduce or eliminate cancer, slow its growth, and reduce the risk of recurrence. Chemotherapy works by targeting cells that are rapidly dividing, which includes cancer cells.

It can also reduce the number of cancer cells in the body, making it easier for other treatments to be more effective.

Chemotherapy also has the potential to reduce the risk of distant metastasis, where cancer cells spread to other parts of the body. By killing cancer cells, chemotherapy can reduce the risk of cancer spreading to other parts of the body.

In addition, chemotherapy can help shrink tumors before surgery. This can make surgery easier and more successful and can reduce the amount of tissue that needs to be removed. Chemotherapy can also help reduce the side effects of radiation therapy, such as fatigue and skin irritation.

Chemotherapy can help reduce the risk of recurrence. By killing cancer cells that may have spread to other parts of the body, chemotherapy can reduce the risk of cancer coming back.

Overall, chemotherapy is an effective treatment for breast cancer and can provide many benefits, including reducing the risk of metastasis, shrinking tumors before surgery, reducing the side effects of radiation therapy, and reducing the risk of recurrence.

The major side effects of chemotherapy treatment for breast cancer

Chemotherapy is a type of treatment used to destroy cancer cells. It works by targeting rapidly dividing cells, which is why it is so effective at killing cancer cells. However, it can also affect healthy cells that divide quickly such as hair follicles and cells in the bone marrow, causing several side effects.

Common side effects of chemotherapy for breast cancer include fatigue, hair loss, nausea, vomiting, diarrhea, and increased risk of infection.

Fatigue: Chemotherapy treatments can be tiring and can cause extreme fatigue. This fatigue can last for several days or weeks after treatment, and it can affect your daily activities.

Hair loss: Hair loss is a common side effect of chemotherapy and can be one of the most distressing. It usually occurs 2–3 weeks after the first treatment and can affect your scalp, eyebrows and eyelashes, and other body hair.

Nausea and vomiting: Nausea and vomiting usually start within a few hours of treatment and can last for several days. Anti-nausea medications can help reduce these side effects.

Diarrhea: Diarrhea is another common side effect of chemotherapy and can cause dehydration, abdominal cramps, and weight loss. Anti-diarrheal medications can help manage this side effect.

Increased risk of infection: Chemotherapy treatments can weaken the immune system and increase the risk of infection. People receiving chemotherapy should take extra precautions to avoid getting sick, such as washing their hands often and avoiding contact with people who are sick.

These are the most common side effects of chemotherapy for breast cancer. However, other side effects can occur, so it is important to talk to your doctor about any changes in your health.

Complementary and Alternative Therapy

Complementary therapies

Complementary therapies are nontraditional treatments that may be used in combination with traditional medicine to help treat breast cancer. These therapies may include massage, acupuncture, yoga, meditation, and other mindfulness-based practices, as well as dietary and lifestyle changes.

Massage therapy can help improve sleep and reduce stress, which can be beneficial for people with breast cancer. Massage can also help reduce pain and improve circulation, which can help with the side effects of chemotherapy and radiation.

Acupuncture is believed to promote the flow of energy and balance the body's qi, or life force. Acupuncture may help reduce fatigue, pain, and nausea, and may also help reduce anxiety and depression.

Yoga and meditation can help reduce stress and anxiety, and may also help improve physical strength and flexibility. Both practices can also help with insomnia and fatigue, which are common side effects of breast cancer and its treatment.

Dietary and lifestyle changes can also be beneficial for people with breast cancer. Eating a balanced diet, exercising regularly, and getting enough sleep can help reduce stress and boost the immune system. Quitting smoking and reducing alcohol consumption can also help reduce the risk of breast cancer recurrence.

Alternative therapy

Alternative therapies for the treatment of breast cancer are treatments that are not part of conventional cancer care, such as surgery, chemotherapy, radiation, and hormone therapy. These treatments are not widely accepted by the medical community and are usually not covered by insurance. Examples of alternative therapies for breast cancer include:

• Acupuncture: This ancient Chinese practice uses the insertion of thin needles into specific points on the body to relieve pain and stimulate healing.

• Aromatherapy: The use of essential oils from plants to reduce stress, boost immunity, and support healing.

• Herbal medicine: The use of herbs and plants to treat diseases and ailments.

• Hypnotherapy: The use of hypnosis to help induce relaxation, reduce anxiety, and promote healing.

• Meditation: The practice of calming the mind and body through mindfulness and relaxation techniques.

• Nutrition and diet: The use of food and supplements to support the body's natural healing processes.

• Yoga: The practice of stretching, breathing, and meditation to reduce stress and promote physical and mental well-being.

These alternative therapies are not meant to replace conventional cancer therapies, but rather to complement and support them.

It is important to talk to your doctor about any alternative therapies you are considering, as some may interfere with the effectiveness of traditional treatments.

CHAPTER 4

Nutrition and Breast Cancer

Nutrition plays a role in the prevention of breast cancer, as well as the overall health of those who have already been diagnosed. Eating a balanced diet with plenty of fruits, vegetables, and whole grains is important for overall health, as well as reducing the risk of breast cancer.

Fruits and vegetables contain many antioxidants, which help to reduce inflammation and damage to cells. These antioxidants can help protect against certain forms of cancer, including breast cancer. Whole grains contain fiber, which is important for digestion and can help reduce the risk of certain cancers.

Studies have also found that certain foods, such as red meat and processed meats, are associated with an increased risk of breast cancer. Limiting the intake of these foods can help reduce the risk. Eating a diet high in plant-based foods, such as fruits and vegetables, is important for overall health and reducing the risk of breast cancer.

In addition to a healthy diet, staying active and maintaining a healthy weight are also important for reducing the risk of breast cancer.

Limit alcohol intake: Drinking alcohol can increase the risk of breast cancer. Women who drink even small amounts of alcohol should limit their intake to no more than one drink per day.

Maintain a healthy weight: Being overweight or obese can increase your risk of breast cancer. Eating a healthy diet and exercising regularly can help you maintain a healthy weight.

Nutrition for breast cancer treatment

Nutrition is an important component of breast cancer treatment. A healthy diet can help support the body during the treatment process and help reduce the risk of recurrence and other complications.

Good nutrition can help prevent or reduce side effects associated with breast cancer treatment such as nausea, diarrhea, constipation, and fatigue. Eating a balanced diet that includes a variety of foods is important for overall health.

A diet that is high in fresh fruits and vegetables, lean proteins, and whole grains can help reduce the risk of recurrence and other health complications. Eating a balanced diet can also help to provide the body with the vitamins, minerals, and antioxidants it needs to fight cancer and support the body's natural healing process.

It is important to eat a variety of foods and avoid processed and refined foods. Eating a balanced diet that includes a variety of foods can help to ensure that the body gets the nutrients it needs to stay healthy and fight cancer. Eating a variety of healthy foods can also provide the body with the energy it needs to cope with the stress of cancer treatment.

Healthy diet for treating breast cancer

1. Eating a healthy diet is a key part of breast cancer treatment and recovery. It is important to eat a balanced diet that is rich in fruits and vegetables, whole grains, and lean proteins. Additionally, limiting processed and sugary foods can help to reduce inflammation and support the body's natural healing processes.

2. Eating adequate amounts of fruits and vegetables can help to give the body the essential vitamins, minerals, and antioxidants it needs to fight off cancer cells. Fruits and vegetables are also rich in fiber, which can help to reduce the risk of breast cancer recurrence and improve overall health.

3. Whole grains are also an important part of a healthy diet for breast cancer treatment. Whole grains provide essential vitamins and minerals and have been linked to a lower risk of cancer recurrence. Additionally, whole grains can help to keep blood sugar levels stable, preventing unhealthy spikes and dips in energy levels.

4. Lean proteins are also beneficial for breast cancer treatment. Lean proteins provide essential amino acids that help to build and repair cells in the body. Additionally, lean proteins can help to reduce

inflammation, which is a key factor in cancer development and recurrence.

5. Eating healthy fats is also important for breast cancer treatment. such as those found in fish, nuts, and vegetable oils, are considered healthy and can help reduce the risk of breast cancer.

Breast Cancer Cook Book

Cookbook for the treatment of breast cancer

1. Curried Lentil Soup: Curried lentil soup is a healthy and flavorful soup that is packed with nutrition. It is also a great source of plant-based protein, which is important for people with breast cancer. The soup itself is made with lentils, curry powder, and a variety of vegetables. It is a very easy and quick meal to prepare and can be enjoyed hot or cold. Lentils are a great source of dietary fiber, which helps keep the body regular and aids in digestion. The curry powder has anti-inflammatory properties, which can help reduce inflammation associated with breast cancer. Additionally, vegetables provide essential vitamins and minerals, which can help the body stay healthy and fight off cancer.

2. Spaghetti Squash with Marinara Sauce: Spaghetti squash is a healthy and versatile vegetable that is a great addition to any meal. It has a mild, sweet flavor, and when cooked, its flesh easily separates into thin, spaghetti-like strands. When served with marinara sauce, it is a great source of plant-based protein, vitamins, minerals, and dietary fiber. The marinara sauce adds a delicious flavor to the spaghetti squash and is also full of antioxidants, which can help fight off cancer cells.

3. Broccoli and Tofu Stir-Fry: Broccoli and tofu stir-fry is a flavorful and nutritious meal that is great for people with breast cancer. Broccoli is a cruciferous vegetable that is packed with vitamins, minerals, and dietary fiber. It is also a great source of anti-cancer compounds, such as sulforaphane, which can help fight off cancer cells. Tofu is a plant-based protein that is low in calories and fat and is a great addition to any meal. When these two ingredients are stir-fried together, they create a delicious dish that is full of flavor and nutrition.

4. Baked Salmon with Vegetables: Baked salmon is a healthy and flavorful dish that is full of essential nutrients. Salmon is a great source of omega-3 fatty

acids, which can help reduce inflammation associated with breast cancer. It is also a great source of protein, which is essential for people with cancer. When served with a variety of vegetables, such as broccoli, carrots, and bell peppers, it creates a balanced meal that is full of vitamins, minerals, and dietary fiber. This meal is also very easy to prepare and can be enjoyed hot or cold.

Healthy drinks for the treatment of breast cancer

1. Green tea: Green tea is rich in antioxidants, which help to reduce the risk of breast cancer. Studies have found that women who drank at least one cup of green tea a day had a 22 percent lower risk of developing breast cancer. The antioxidants in green tea may help to reduce inflammation, which can help to protect against cancer.

2. Turmeric: Turmeric is a powerful antioxidant that has been found to reduce the growth of cancer cells in some studies. It may also help to reduce inflammation and boost the immune system, which can help to prevent cancer.

3. Ginger: Ginger has anti-inflammatory and antioxidant properties, which can help to reduce the risk of cancer. Studies have found that women who frequently consumed ginger tea had a significantly reduced risk of developing breast cancer.

4. Pomegranate: Pomegranates are rich in antioxidants and may help to reduce the risk of cancer. Studies have found that the antioxidants in pomegranates can help to reduce the growth of cancer cells.

5. Beetroot: Beetroots are packed with antioxidants and other nutrients, which can help to reduce the risk of cancer. Studies have found that women who regularly consumed beetroot juice had a significantly reduced risk of developing breast cancer.

Breakfast Combinations for Breast Cancer Treatment

1. Oatmeal with Berries and Almonds: Oatmeal is a high-fiber food that helps reduce the risk of breast cancer. Berries are rich in antioxidants that help protect the body from cancer-causing free radicals. Almonds are high in healthy monounsaturated fat and fiber, both of which have been linked to a lower risk of breast cancer.

2. Whole Wheat Toast with Avocado and Tomatoes: Whole wheat toast is a good source of complex carbohydrates, which can help reduce the risk of breast cancer. Avocados are high in healthy monounsaturated fats that can help reduce inflammation, a known risk factor for breast cancer. Tomatoes are a rich source of lycopene, an antioxidant that helps protect the body from damaging free radicals.

3. Greek Yogurt with Walnuts and Honey: Greek yogurt is a good source of protein and calcium, both of which can help reduce the risk of breast cancer. Walnuts are high in omega-3 fatty acids, which have been linked to a lower risk of breast cancer.

Honey is high in antioxidants and anti-inflammatory compounds, which can help protect the body from cancer-causing free radicals.

4. Egg and Vegetable Scramble: Eggs are a good source of high-quality protein and choline, both of which have been linked to a lower risk of breast cancer. Vegetables are rich in antioxidants and phytochemicals, which can help protect the body from cancer-causing free radicals.

5. Whole Wheat Pancakes with Almond Butter and Berries: Whole wheat pancakes are a good source of complex carbohydrates, which can help reduce the risk of breast cancer. Almond butter is a good source of healthy monounsaturated fat and fiber, both of which have been linked to a lower risk of breast cancer. Berries are high in antioxidants that help protect the body from cancer-causing free radicals.

6. Brown Rice and Bean Bowl: Brown rice is a good source of complex carbohydrates, which can help reduce the risk of breast cancer. Beans are a good source of protein and fiber, both of which have been linked to a lower risk of breast cancer.

7. Quinoa Bowl with Avocado and Tomatoes: Quinoa is a high-fiber food that helps reduce the risk of breast cancer. Avocado is a good source of healthy monounsaturated fat and fiber, both of which have been linked to a lower risk of breast cancer. Tomatoes are rich in lycopene, an antioxidant that helps protect the body from damaging free radicals.

8. Omelet with Spinach and Mushrooms: Eggs are a good source of high-quality protein and choline, both of which have been linked to a lower risk of breast cancer. Spinach is rich in antioxidants and phytochemicals, which can help protect the body from cancer-causing free radicals. Mushrooms are high in selenium, which has been linked to a lower risk of breast cancer.

9. Smoothie with Kefir and Berries: Kefir is a good source of probiotics, which can help reduce inflammation, a known risk factor for breast cancer. Berries are high in antioxidants that help protect the body from cancer-causing free radicals.

10. Oatmeal with Chia Seeds and Apples: Oatmeal is a high-fiber food that helps reduce the risk of breast cancer. Apples are rich in antioxidants that help protect the body from damaging free radicals.

Lunch combinations for Breast Cancer Treatment

1. Salmon with Green Beans and Brown Rice: This combination is rich in omega-3 fatty acids, which have been linked to breast cancer prevention. Brown rice is a good source of fiber, which helps to lower levels of estrogen in the body, and green beans are a great source of vitamins and minerals that can help keep cells healthy.

2. Kale and Quinoa Salad: Kale is a great source of indole-3-carbinol, a compound that helps to reduce the risk of breast cancer. Quinoa is a complete protein, containing all nine essential amino acids, and is also high in fiber, making it beneficial for reducing estrogen levels.

3. Lentil Soup with Carrots and Onions: Lentils are a great source of fiber, protein, and other vitamins and minerals that can help reduce the risk of breast cancer.

The combination of carrots and onions provides additional antioxidants and phytochemicals to further lower the risk of cancer.

4. Baked Sweet Potato with Avocado: Sweet potatoes are high in antioxidants, which can help reduce the risk of breast cancer. The inclusion of avocado adds healthy fats, which can help reduce inflammation and the risk of cancer.

5. Chickpea and Spinach Curry: Chickpeas are a great source of fiber and protein, both of which have been linked to reduced risk of breast cancer. The addition of spinach provides additional vitamins and minerals to further reduce the risk.

6. Turkey and Broccoli Stir-Fry: Lean proteins, such as turkey, have been linked to reduced risk of breast cancer. The addition of broccoli adds additional vitamins, minerals, and antioxidants to further reduce the risk.

7. Cauliflower and Brown Rice Bowl: Cauliflower is rich in antioxidants, which can help reduce the risk of breast cancer. The addition of brown rice provides a good source of fiber to help reduce estrogen levels.

8. Soup with Beans and Vegetables: Beans are a great source of fiber, protein, and other vitamins and minerals that can help reduce the risk of breast cancer. The combination of vegetables provides additional antioxidants and phytochemicals to further reduce the risk.

9. Tofu and Broccoli: Tofu is a great source of plant-based protein and contains isoflavones, which have been linked to reduced risk of breast cancer. The addition of broccoli adds additional vitamins, minerals, and antioxidants to further reduce the risk.

10. Egg and Spinach Salad: Eggs are a great source of protein and omega-3 fatty acids, both of which have been linked to reduced risk of breast cancer. The addition of spinach provides additional vitamins and minerals to further reduce the risk.

Dinner Combinations for Breast Cancer Treatment

1. Grilled Salmon with Asparagus: Salmon is a rich source of omega-3 fatty acids, which are believed to help reduce the risk of breast cancer. Asparagus is high in folate, which helps protect DNA and cells from damage that could lead to cancer.

2. Mushroom Stir-Fry with Broccoli: Broccoli is a cruciferous vegetable that contains compounds that may reduce the risk of breast cancer. Mushrooms are also rich in antioxidants that may help reduce the risk of cancer.

3. Lentil Soup with Spinach: Lentils are a great source of fiber and plant-based protein, both of which may help reduce the risk of breast cancer. Spinach is also high in antioxidants, which may help protect against cancer.

4. Tofu and Vegetable Stir-Fry: Tofu is a great source of plant-based protein and contains isoflavones, which may help reduce the risk of breast cancer.

Stir-frying a mix of vegetables is also a great way to get lots of cancer-fighting antioxidants.

5. Baked Salmon with Kale: Baked salmon is a great source of omega-3 fatty acids and kale is packed with antioxidants. Both may help reduce the risk of breast cancer.

6. Quinoa with Roasted Vegetables: Quinoa is a great source of protein and contains many antioxidants that may help reduce the risk of breast cancer. Roasting vegetables brings out their flavor and helps to retain some of their cancer-fighting compounds.

7. Lentil Salad with Tomatoes: Lentils are a great source of fiber and plant-based protein, which may help reduce the risk of breast cancer. Tomatoes are high in the antioxidant lycopene, which may also help reduce the risk of cancer.

8. Turkey Burger with Sweet Potato Fries: Turkey is a lean source of protein and sweet potatoes are high in antioxidants. Both may help reduce the risk of breast cancer.

9. Grilled Veggie Sandwich with Hummus: Grilling vegetables bring out their flavor and help to retain some of their cancer-fighting compounds. Hummus is a great source of fiber and plant-based protein, which may help reduce the risk of breast cancer.

Dessert Combinations for Breast Cancer Treatment

1. Carrot Cake and Blueberry Smoothie: Carrot cake is high in beta-carotene, which is a potent antioxidant that can help prevent cancer cell growth. Blueberries are also packed with antioxidants, which can help fight off the free radicals that can cause cancer cell growth.

2. Oatmeal and Cranberry Juice: Oatmeal is a good source of fiber which helps support the digestive tract and can help reduce the risk of cancer.

Cranberry juice is also high in antioxidants, which can help fight off cancer cells.

3. Apple Pie and Green Tea: Apples are a good source of both soluble and insoluble fiber, which can help reduce the risk of cancer. Green tea is packed with antioxidants that can help fight off the free radicals that can cause cancer cells to form.

4. Chocolate Cake and Pomegranate Juice: Chocolate cake is high in antioxidants, which can help fight off cancer cells. Pomegranate juice is also high in antioxidants, which can help reduce the risk of cancer.

5. Strawberry Shortcake and Red Wine: Strawberries are a good source of both soluble and insoluble fiber, which can help reduce the risk of cancer. Red wine is also high in antioxidants, which can help fight off cancer cells.

6. Mango and Yogurt Parfait: Mangoes are high in antioxidants, which can help reduce the risk of cancer. Yogurt is also a good source of probiotics, which can help support the digestive tract and can help reduce the risk of cancer.

7. Bananas Foster and Acai Juice: Bananas are a good source of both soluble and insoluble fiber, which can help reduce the risk of cancer. Acai juice is also high in antioxidants, which can help fight off cancer cells.

8. Cheesecake and Green Juice: Cheesecake is high in calcium, which can help reduce the risk of cancer. Green juice is also high in antioxidants, which can help fight off cancer cells.

9. Key Lime Pie and Turmeric Tea: Key limes are high in antioxidants, which can help reduce the risk of cancer. Turmeric tea is also high in antioxidants, which can help fight off cancer cells.

10. Pineapple Upside-Down Cake and Ginger Tea: Pineapple is a good source of both soluble and insoluble fiber, which can help reduce the risk of cancer. Ginger tea is also high in antioxidants, which can help fight off cancer cells.

CHAPTER 5

Lifestyle and Breast Cancer

Stress and Breast Cancer

Stress has been linked to an increased risk of developing breast cancer. High levels of stress can cause the body to release hormones that can damage cells and weaken the immune system, making it harder for the body to fight off cancer. Stress can also lead to unhealthy lifestyle choices like smoking and poor diet, which can increase the risk of developing breast cancer. Additionally, stress can lead to sleep deprivation, which has been linked to an increased risk of cancer.

It is important to manage stress levels to reduce the risk of cancer. This can be done by engaging in activities like yoga, meditation, and regular exercise. Additionally, maintaining a healthy diet, getting good sleep, and making time for yourself can help reduce stress.

Managing stress for the treatment of breast cancer

Stress is a normal part of life, but it can have a significant impact on physical and mental well-being, especially when it comes to treating breast cancer. Stress can interfere with treatment, increase inflammation in the body, and weaken the immune system.

Managing stress is an important part of breast cancer treatment. There are several ways to reduce stress and promote relaxation, including:

• Exercise: Regular physical activity can help reduce stress by releasing endorphins, which are the body's natural feel-good hormones.

• Meditation and relaxation: Meditation and relaxation techniques can help you find a sense of inner peace, reduce stress, and improve your overall well-being.

• Healthy diet: Eating a healthy diet may help reduce the physical effects of stress by providing your body with the nutrients it needs.

• Support groups: Joining a support group can provide you with a safe space to share your thoughts and feelings with people who understand what you're going through.

• Therapy: Talking to a therapist or counselor can help you learn how to manage stress and cope with the emotions associated with breast cancer treatment.

• Make sure to get enough rest, practice self-care activities like yoga or massage, and do things that bring you joy.

Managing stress is an important part of breast cancer treatment. By taking steps to reduce stress and take care of your physical, mental, and emotional well-being, you can help ensure that you are getting the most out of your treatment and recovery.

Exercise and Breast Cancer

Exercise has been shown to have significant benefits for individuals with breast cancer, both during and after treatment.

Regular physical activity can reduce symptoms associated with breast cancer and help people to manage the side effects of treatments. It can also help to reduce the risk of recurrence and improve overall physical and mental health.

Exercise can help to reduce fatigue, improve sleep and reduce anxiety and depression. It can also improve overall physical functioning and reduce the risk of lymphedema, a condition that can occur after breast cancer treatment in which fluid builds up in the arm.

In addition, exercise can help to improve cardiovascular health and reduce the risk of other chronic diseases. Studies have shown that regular physical activity can lower the risk of breast cancer recurrence and improve overall survival. Exercise can also help to maintain and improve bone health and reduce the risk of fractures.

Regular exercise can help to improve body image and self-esteem, which can be important for individuals who have undergone surgery or other treatments for breast cancer. In addition, physical activity can help to promote a positive attitude, which can be beneficial during treatment and recovery.

Exercise that helps in the treatment of breast cancer

Exercise is an important part of any breast cancer treatment plan. Studies have found that physical activity can reduce the risk of breast cancer recurrence and mortality, as well as improve quality of life.

Aerobic exercise: Regular aerobic exercise can help reduce fatigue, improve energy levels, and reduce stress and anxiety. Aerobic activities such as walking, jogging, cycling, swimming, or dancing can help with recovery from breast cancer treatment.

Strength training: Strength training can help improve muscle strength and endurance, which may be affected by chemotherapy or radiation. Resistance exercises such as weight lifting, yoga, and Pilates can help improve physical strength.

Yoga: Yoga can help reduce stress, improve mental clarity, and reduce fatigue.

Tai chi: Tai chi is a form of exercise that combines slow, gentle movements with meditation and breathing.

Pilates: Pilates is a form of exercise that combines strengthening and stretching exercises with breathing and mental focus. It can help improve flexibility, balance, and core strength.

Stretching: Stretching can help reduce fatigue and improve flexibility and range of motion. Gentle stretching exercises such as yoga, tai chi, and Pilates can help improve overall physical well-being.

Diet and Breast Cancer

A diet high in plant-based foods is linked to a reduced risk of breast cancer. Plant-based foods are rich in fiber, vitamins, and minerals, which may help protect against the disease. Research suggests that a diet high in fruits, vegetables, whole grains, and legumes may reduce the risk of breast cancer. Additionally, plant-based foods are naturally low in fat, which may also help reduce the risk.

In addition to reducing the risk of breast cancer, a plant-based diet can also help improve overall health.

Plant-based foods are a good source of vitamins, minerals, and antioxidants, which can help improve immune system health and reduce the risk of other chronic diseases. Additionally, plant-based foods are naturally lower in calories and fat than animal-based foods, making them a good choice for weight loss or maintaining a healthy weight.

Importance of plant-based food in the treatment of breast cancer

Plant-based foods have been found to have a beneficial role in the treatment of breast cancer. Studies have shown that consuming a diet high in plant-based foods can reduce the risk of developing certain types of breast cancer, as well as reduce the risk of cancer recurrence and mortality.

Studies have found that diets rich in whole grains, legumes, fruits, and vegetables are associated with a lower risk of breast cancer and mortality.

Whole grains, legumes, and vegetables are high in fiber, which helps reduce inflammation and can help protect against cancer. Fruits and vegetables are also rich in antioxidants, which can help fight oxidative damage in the body and reduce the risk of cancer.

In addition, plant-based foods are rich in phytochemicals, which are compounds found in plant foods that may protect against cancer growth and progression. Phytochemicals such as isoflavones and polyphenols, which are found in soy products, have been found to have protective effects against certain types of breast cancer.

Plant-based foods are also high in vitamins and minerals, which can help support the immune system and reduce the risk of breast cancer. For example, folate, which is found in leafy green vegetables, has been found to reduce the risk of breast cancer. Vitamin D, which is found in certain plant foods, has also been found to reduce the risk of breast cancer.

The scientific evidence for the benefits of a plant-based diet in the treatment of breast cancer is strong.

Consuming a diet high in plant-based foods can reduce the risk of developing certain types of breast cancer, as well as reduce the risk of cancer recurrence and mortality. Eating a diet rich in fruits and vegetables, whole grains, legumes, and healthy fats can help support the immune system and reduce the risk of breast cancer.

CHAPTER 6

Managing Side Effect

Pain and Fatigue

Pain management

Pain is a common symptom experienced by people living with breast cancer. Pain can range from mild to severe and can be caused by cancer itself, treatment side effects, and the disease's progression.

Pain management strategies include:

• Medication: Over-the-counter and prescription medications, such as non-steroidal anti-inflammatory drugs (NSAIDs) and opioids, can be used to help manage pain.

• Physical therapy: Physical therapy can help reduce pain by helping to improve flexibility, strength, and range of motion.

• Acupuncture: Acupuncture can help reduce pain by stimulating the body's natural pain-relieving endorphins.

• Heat and cold therapy: Applying hot or cold packs to the affected area can help reduce pain.

• Relaxation techniques: Relaxation techniques, such as deep breathing, progressive muscle relaxation, and guided imagery, can help reduce pain.

• Complementary therapies: Complementary therapies, such as massage, aromatherapy, and yoga, can help reduce pain.

Fatigue management

Fatigue is a common symptom experienced by people living with breast cancer. It is caused by cancer itself, treatment side effects, and the disease's progression.

Fatigue management strategies include:

1. Exercise: Regular physical activity can help reduce fatigue and improve overall function. Light aerobic exercise, such as walking, can be beneficial for cancer-related fatigue.

2. Sleep: Ensuring adequate sleep can help reduce fatigue. Establishing a regular sleep routine can help with this.

3. Diet: Eating a nutritious diet can help combat fatigue. Eating a balanced diet with plenty of fruits and vegetables is recommended.

4. Stress Management: Stress can worsen fatigue. Relaxation techniques such as meditation, yoga, and deep breathing can help reduce stress and improve fatigue.

5. Support Groups: Joining a support group can provide social support and help cancer patients cope with fatigue.

6. Acupuncture: Acupuncture may help reduce fatigue in some people.

7. Energy Conservation: Conserving energy can help reduce fatigue. This may include pacing activities and taking frequent rest breaks.

8. Cognitive Behavioral Therapy: Cognitive behavioral therapy can help cancer patients develop coping strategies for managing fatigue.

Nausea and Vomiting

Nausea and vomiting are common side effects of breast cancer treatment. While they can be unpleasant and disruptive, there are ways to manage them.

The management of these symptoms is important for improving quality of life and avoiding further complications.

The most effective approach to managing nausea and vomiting caused by breast cancer treatments is to use a combination of medications and lifestyle interventions.

Medications: Antiemetic drugs, such as ondansetron and granisetron, can help to control nausea and vomiting. These medications work by blocking the action of serotonin, a chemical in the brain that helps to regulate nausea and vomiting.

Lifestyle interventions: Eating small, frequent meals throughout the day and avoiding strong-smelling and greasy foods can help to reduce nausea. Additionally, avoiding activities that may trigger nausea, such as riding in cars or on amusement park rides, can be beneficial.

Other strategies: Acupuncture and other alternative treatments can also help relieve nausea and vomiting. Additionally, relaxation techniques, such as deep breathing and progressive muscle relaxation, can help to reduce stress and reduce nausea.

Sexuality and Intimacy

Sexuality and intimacy in breast cancer are important areas of management that should be addressed to improve the overall quality of life for patients. Treatment of breast cancer can have a significant impact on a patient's sexual functioning, making it difficult to manage. Here are some strategies to help manage sexuality and intimacy in breast cancer:

1. Communication: Communicating openly with a partner, family, friends, and healthcare providers can help patients feel more supported and provide an avenue for discussing concerns and questions related to sexuality and intimacy.

2. Education: Learning about the various physical and psychological impacts of breast cancer can help patients prepare for and manage changes in their sexuality and intimacy.

3. Self-care: Practicing self-care activities such as exercise, relaxation, and good nutrition can help patients manage stress and improve overall well-being.

4. Psychological counseling: Psychological counseling can help patients explore their feelings, manage anxiety, and build coping skills.

5. Medication: Some medications can help manage the physical side effects of breast cancer treatments, such as pain and fatigue.

6. Sexual aids: There are many sexual aids available that can help make intimacy more enjoyable and comfortable for patients.

7. Alternative treatments: Alternative treatments such as acupuncture and massage can help reduce stress and promote relaxation.

8. Support groups: Joining a support group can provide a safe and supportive environment for patients to discuss their experiences with other people who are going through a similar situation.

Hair Loss

1. Communication with the Medical Team: It is important to discuss any concerns related to hair loss with your medical team so that they can develop a personalized plan to manage hair loss.

2. Wearing a Wig: Wearing a wig can help to reduce the psychological impact of hair loss and provide a sense of normalcy.

3. Scalp Cooling: Scalp cooling is a technique that has been shown to reduce hair loss in some breast cancer patients undergoing chemotherapy.

4. Nutrition: A healthy diet rich in protein, iron, zinc, and biotin can help to promote hair growth.

5. Stress Management: Stress can exacerbate hair loss, so it is important to practice stress management techniques such as yoga, meditation, and relaxation.

6. Topical Treatments: There are a variety of topical treatments that can be used to stimulate hair growth and reduce hair loss.

7. Hair Care: It is important to use gentle hair care techniques and to avoid heat styling and chemical treatments.

8. Support Groups: Joining a support group can provide emotional support for those dealing with hair loss due to breast cancer.

CHAPTER 7

Healthy Living Ever After

Healthy maintenance after the treatment of breast cancer includes lifestyle changes, regular checkups, and medications.

Lifestyle Changes: A healthy lifestyle is essential for a successful recovery after breast cancer treatment. This includes eating a healthy diet, getting regular exercise, and avoiding or limiting alcohol and tobacco. Eating a balanced diet may help reduce the risk of recurrence and other health problems. It is important to focus on whole grains, fruits, vegetables, and lean proteins.

Exercise is important for overall health, and it can also help reduce the risk of recurrence and improve quality of life. Exercise can help reduce fatigue, boost energy levels, and improve mood. Avoiding alcohol and tobacco can help reduce the risk of recurrence and other health problems.

Regular Checkups: After the treatment of breast cancer, it is important to attend regular checkups and screenings. This may include mammograms, physical exams, and blood tests. Regular checkups can help catch any recurrence early and can also help with monitoring for side effects from medications or other treatments.

Medications: After the treatment of breast cancer, medications may be prescribed to help prevent a recurrence. This may include hormone therapy, chemotherapy, targeted therapy, or immunotherapy. The type of medication prescribed will depend on the type of breast cancer and the stage of the disease. It is important to discuss the risks, benefits, and side effects of all medications with your doctor.

Skincare

1. Protect Your Skin From the Sun: Ultraviolet (UV) radiation from the sun and tanning beds can damage your skin and increase your risk of skin cancer. Wear protective clothing, such as long-sleeved shirts and hats, and use a broad-spectrum sunscreen of SPF 30 or higher on exposed skin.

2. Reduce Stress: Cancer treatments such as chemotherapy, radiation, and surgery can be stressful. To help reduce stress, try relaxation techniques such as yoga, deep breathing, or massage.

3. Moisturize: Cancer treatments can make your skin dry and itchy. To reduce dryness and itching, use a moisturizer after washing and bathing. Look for products that are free of fragrances and dyes, which can be drying and irritating.

4. Avoid Skin Irritants: Chemicals and other irritants can dry out and irritate your skin. Avoid products that contain alcohol and fragrances, and use mild soap.

5. Avoid Hot Water: Hot water can dry out your skin, so try taking baths or showers in warm, not hot, water.

6. Clean Your Skin Gently: Over-scrubbing and harsh cleansers can irritate your skin. To clean your skin, use lukewarm water and a gentle, non-soap cleanser.

7. Eat a Healthy Diet: Eating a balanced diet can help keep your skin healthy. Try to include plenty of fruits, vegetables, whole grains, and lean proteins.

8. Try Home Remedies: Natural remedies such as aloe vera, coconut oil, and oatmeal baths can help soothe irritated skin. Talk to your doctor before trying any new home remedies

Skincare routine

A skincare routine after the treatment of breast cancer is an important part of recovery. The skin can become very sensitive after radiation and chemotherapy, and it is important to take care of it.

The first step is to use gentle cleansers and moisturizers. Look for products that are free of fragrances, dyes, and harsh detergents, as these can be irritating to the skin.

It is also important to use sunscreen every day, even on cloudy days, as the skin can be more prone to sunburn and other skin damage.

It is also important to avoid hot showers and baths and to use lukewarm or cool water instead. Hot water can be too harsh on the skin and can cause further irritation. Bathing with colloidal oatmeal can also be beneficial, as it can help soothe and hydrate the skin.

After bathing, it is important to moisturize the skin as soon as possible, as this can help keep the skin hydrated. Choose a moisturizer that is specifically formulated for sensitive skin, as this will be less irritating.

 It is important to protect the skin from extreme temperatures. Wear protective clothing and hats when outside, and avoid using heating pads or electric blankets, as these can be too harsh on the skin.

By following these tips, you can help your skin to heal after breast cancer treatment and keep it healthy and hydrated.

Hair Care

Hair care is an important aspect of cancer treatment and recovery. For those undergoing chemotherapy and radiation, hair loss is an inevitable side effect. It is important to protect the scalp and hair while undergoing treatment and during recovery.

For those undergoing chemotherapy, scalp cooling techniques such as cold caps can be used to reduce the amount of hair loss. These caps are worn during chemotherapy and are cooled to a very low temperature to decrease the number of chemotherapy drugs reaching the scalp and hair follicles.

For those undergoing radiation, the use of a scalp protector is important to protect the scalp from the harsh effects of radiation. There are several types of scalp protectors available, including creams, gels, and sprays. These products contain ingredients such as aloe, beeswax, and shea butter to help protect the scalp and hair from radiation.

It is also important to maintain a healthy diet, adequate hydration, and stress reduction during cancer treatment. Eating a diet rich in antioxidants, such as fruits and vegetables, can help to reduce the amount of hair loss and improve the health of the scalp and hair. Drinking plenty of water helps to keep the scalp and hair hydrated and healthy. Finally, reducing stress and getting enough rest can help to reduce the amount of hair loss.

Once treatment is complete, several strategies can be used to help improve the health of the scalp and hair. Using shampoos and conditioners designed for those who have undergone chemotherapy or radiation can help to restore the scalp and hair. Scalp massages can also help to improve scalp circulation and promote healthy hair growth. Additionally, using natural oils, such as coconut oil, avocado oil, and jojoba oil, can help to nourish the scalp and restore the health of the hair.

Support Groups

Support groups are an invaluable resource for individuals who have been diagnosed and treated for breast cancer. Support groups provide individuals with an opportunity to meet other people who have experienced similar experiences, share stories, and discuss strategies for managing the physical and emotional effects of breast cancer.

Support groups provide a safe, non-judgmental space for individuals to talk openly about the challenges and successes of their breast cancer journey. They can provide a sense of community and belonging, which can help build self-esteem and resiliency. In addition, support groups can provide individuals with access to resources and information, such as coping skills and strategies to help manage their cancer-related stress.

Support groups can also help individuals to connect with others who are facing similar challenges and to gain insight into different ways of dealing with the diagnosis and treatment of breast cancer. They can also provide a platform for individuals to share tips and strategies for managing side effects, such as fatigue and depression.

Finally, support groups can provide a sense of hope and optimism, which can be invaluable for individuals who are struggling to cope with their cancer diagnosis and treatment. By providing a safe space for individuals to connect and share their stories, support groups can help to reduce feelings of isolation and provide a sense of comfort and understanding.

Professional Help

Professional follow-up care is essential after the treatment of breast cancer. Professional follow-up care includes regular check-ups with your doctor, as well as regular monitoring for any physical and emotional changes.

Regular check-ups are important to make sure that the cancer is not coming back. During these check-ups, your doctor will check your body for any lumps or changes in your breasts. They may also do tests such as mammograms and MRIs to check for any signs of recurrence.

Regular monitoring of physical and emotional changes is also important. After treatment, some people may notice physical changes, such as fatigue, pain, or changes in their skin. It is important to keep track of any changes and talk to your doctor about them.

It is also important to monitor your emotional health. Cancer treatment can be a difficult experience, and some people may experience depression, anxiety, or other mental health issues. It is important to talk to a mental health professional about these issues and get help if needed.

 It is important to stay in touch with your doctor. Your doctor can provide support and guidance throughout your recovery, as well as answer any questions or concerns you may have.

Professional follow-up care is essential after treatment for breast cancer. It is important to stay in contact with your doctor and to monitor your physical and emotional health. If any changes or concerns arise, it is important to talk to your doctor or seek help from a mental health professional.

Moving forward with life

1. Establish a New Routine

After finishing breast cancer treatment, it can be difficult to adjust to a life without appointments and check-ups. It is important to establish a new routine that includes healthy lifestyle habits, such as regular exercise and nutritious eating. Not only will this routine help you maintain your physical health, but it can also provide a sense of normalcy and structure.

2. Connect with Others

Connecting with others who have gone through a similar experience can be a great source of support. Joining a support group or attending a breast cancer retreat can provide invaluable resources and help you feel less alone. Take advantage of online forums and resources to stay connected with other survivors and find support.

3. Take Time for Yourself

Surviving breast cancer can take a toll on your physical and emotional health. Taking time for yourself and engaging in activities that bring you joy can help you stay positive and cope with any lingering anxiety or depression. Find some time each day to do something you enjoy, such as reading, journaling, listening to music, or taking a walk.

4. Set Realistic Goals

It is important to set realistic goals for yourself and focus on taking things one step at a time. Celebrate small successes and understand that it is ok to take a break when you need it. Having a plan and setting achievable goals can help you stay motivated and continue to move forward.

5. Stay Informed

Stay informed about the latest research and treatments related to breast cancer. This will help you stay up-to-date on the latest developments and better understand any changes or symptoms that may arise. It is also important to talk to your doctor about any questions or concerns you may have.

6. Seek Support: Don't forget that you have a support system of family, friends, and healthcare providers who can help you adjust to life beyond breast cancer treatment. Reach out to them for help and advice as needed.

7. Find Purpose: Look for ways to use your experiences to help others. Whether it's connecting with other breast cancer survivors or volunteering in your community, finding purpose can help you stay motivated.

8. Make Self-Care a Priority: Self-care is essential for recovery and wellness after breast cancer treatment. Taking time for yourself and engaging in activities that promote physical, emotional, and mental wellbeing can help you move forward in life and adjust to the changes that have taken place. Examples of self-care activities include meditation, yoga, journaling, exercise, and getting adequate rest.

9. Connect with a Support Network: Having a solid support system is an important part of the recovery

process. Reach out to family and friends and find a support group of other breast cancer survivors to talk to. Being able to share your experiences and feelings with others who understand can help you cope and find the strength to move forward.

10. Create a Positive Mindset: It can be helpful to focus on the positive aspects of your life and practice gratitude. A positive mindset can help bring a sense of peace and happiness, and it can also help to reduce stress and anxiety. Consider making time each day to reflect on the things you are grateful for and focus on the good in your life.

11. Make Healthy Lifestyle Choices: Eating a balanced diet and engaging in regular physical activity can help to promote emotional and physical health. Aim to make healthy lifestyle choices that will help you feel better and have more energy.

Conclusion

The book Knockdown That Breast Cancer is a comprehensive guide to breast cancer awareness, prevention, and treatment. The book provides readers with an in-depth look at the disease and its many stages, from diagnosis and treatment to recovery and long-term care. It also provides practical advice and support for women facing a diagnosis of breast cancer.

The book's conclusion provides readers with a hopeful and inspiring message: that breast cancer can be beaten. It emphasizes the need for early detection, the importance of staying informed about the disease, and the power of positive thinking.
The book's conclusion is a reminder that breast cancer is not an automatic death sentence and that, with the right information and support, women can beat the disease. It is an uplifting message of hope, and a reminder that breast cancer is a fight worth fighting.

www.ingramcontent.com/pod-product-compliance
Lightning Source LLC
Chambersburg PA
CBHW050816250726
48653CB00006B/2247